AIR FRYER COOKBOOK FOR BEGINNERS 2021:

Quick & Easy Recipes. Create Amazing Meals with your Air Fryer.

Tom Smith

CONTENTS

Introduction..ii

What is an Air Fryer?..9

Breakfast Recipes..20

    Cushioned Cheesy Omelet..20

    Crust-Less Quiche..22

    Chorizo Risotto..24

    Egg Yolks With Squid..26

    Parsnip Hash Browns..28

    Very Berry Breakfast Puffs..30

    Milky Scrambled Eggs...32

    Toasties and Sausage in Egg Pond..34

    Banana Bread...36

    Flavorful Bacon Cups..38

Lunch Recipes..40

    Yogurt Garlic Chicken..40

    Lemony Parmesan Salmon...43

    Easiest Tuna Cobbler Ever..45

    Homemade Pork Buns..47

    Chili Bell Peppers Stew...48

Grilled Ham & Cheese...49

Thyme Green Beans...51

Rosemary Lamb..52

Meat Bake...53

Mouthwatering Tuna Melts...54

Poultry Recipes...56

Creamy Coconut Chicken...56

Chinese Chicken Wings..57

Herbed Chicken...58

Chicken Parmesan...59

Mexican Chicken..61

Creamy Chicken, Rice and Peas...62

Prune-stuffed Turkey Tenderloins..64

Sweet & Sour Chicken Thighs..66

Oregano And Lemon Chicken Drumsticks...................................68

Paprika-cumin Rubbed Chicken Tenderloin................................69

Fish and Seafood Recipe...72

Cajun Style Shrimp..72

Crab Cakes..74

Tuna Pie..70

Tuna Puff Pastry..72

Cajun Style Catfish...74

Meat Recipes...76

Lime Lamb Mix..76

Lamb and Corn..77

Herbed Beef and Squash...78

Smoked Beef Mix..80

Marjoram Pork Mix...81

Nutmeg Lamb...82

Greek Beef Mix...83

Beef and Fennel..84

Side Dish Recipes...85

Easy Polenta Pie...85

Bean and Rice Dish...87

Cheesy Potato Mash Casserole..89

Simple Squash Casserole...90

Delicious Ginger Pork Lasagna...92

Baked Sweet Potatoes...94

Broccoli Pasta...95

Cauliflower Rice..96

Refried Beans...98

Sweet Brussels Sprouts...99

Dessert Recipes..100

Fiesta Pastries...100

Classic Buttermilk Biscuits...102

Blueberry bowls..104

Carrot brownies..105

Yogurt cake..106

Chocolate ramekins...107

Grapes cake..108

Carrots bread...109

Pear pudding..110

Lime cake...111

Pear stew...112

Introduction

We as a whole know it, and you are here because you know it as well; practicing good eating habits isn't just a craze decision however a whole change to your way of life and perspective.

Every day you should endeavor to use sound judgment and make child strides towards your wellness objectives. Gradually, you appear to make sound propensities that stick.

In any case, on the planet, we live in today, there is in a real sense enticement everywhere. From the treats bowl at work to the café menu to the inexpensive food joint impeccably positioned on your drive home, it is difficult to deny such flavorful temptations. Anyway, how could one strengthen themselves to keep focused?

We will handle the absolute best tips to help you in accomplishing your wellness objectives, regardless of whether you wish to shed some overabundance fat or are simply needing to look and feel somewhat better, there is consistently an approach to safeguard yourself against undesirable allurements.

Eat before you go

It is hard to settle on solid choices when your stomach is snarling.

Ensure you eat before you head to work, to the store, or any place where you may be directed to settle on a helpless decision in food.

Or then again, take a sound nibble with you. On the off chance that you are continually allowing yourself to quit wasting the time of "hangry-ness," you are obtrusively setting yourself up to eat in the place where there are low-quality nourishments.

It is additionally critical to eat predictable dinners for the day to help you keep focused also. Figure out how to cook in the solace of your own home as opposed to squandering your well-deserved cash on food that truly sometimes falls short for you well. Plan ahead

It is to your greatest advantage to be readied. Start every week by making yourself a dinner plan. Rundown what you need and make it an objective to stick as close as possible to this arrangement. This will assist you with diminishing the occasions you go to the store, which brings about a lessening of hasty purchases.

Plan for eating out as well! Numerous eateries presently post their whole menu online for clients to take a gander at. Understand what alternatives they have accessible, which will settle on it simpler to settle on better choices.

Stunt what triggers you

We all have a form of kryptonite, that delightful yet terrible for-you eats that leave us feeling defenseless and unfit to retaliate.

Keep such enticements out of the picture and therefore irrelevant, or even better, out of your home and office through and through.

To continue through to the end of turning into a better form of yourself, you should get familiar with the significance of settling on choices when faced with better options in contrast to what you are set off by to balance them.

For instance, on the off chance that you resemble me, frozen yogurt is consistently a losing fight. Rather than making a beeline for scoop some mint chocolate chip that is stacked with sugar and incalculable calories, select to make a better form, like Banana Ice Cream!

Research desires

At the point when you end up in a craving for something upsetting for your body, pause for a minute to pause and wonder why you are wanting a specific thing. Would it be what you are wanting? There are large numbers of us, myself notwithstanding, that misunderstanding our enthusiastic longings with food, and unfortunately, food won't ever make up for this sort of shortcoming.

If you are continually succumbing to a type of allurement, look inside yourself and consider what your energy resembles and what you are feeling and thinking at that point. Individuals are more inclined to unfortunate and indulging when they are worried, drained, restless, exhausted, or attempting to adapt to a questionable circumstance. Rather than utilizing food to adapt, assess your passionate status and perceive how you can resolve the antagonism that is filling your awful decision-making with regards to what you eat and what you desire.

Make a way to progress

Focus on it to stay aware of a food diary. Track what you eat, how you feel when you eat things, what causes you to ache for specific things, and so on Regularly, essentially writing down a horrendous decision of food can lead you to settle on much better choices later on.

You can likewise work out mantras in this diary too. Make up an expression you can undoubtedly recollect that will assist you with discovering the inspiration to continue to push ahead in a sound example.

"I'm great."

"I'm taking a stab at extreme wellbeing."

"I'm in charge of the decisions I make."

Follow up on "give-ins" with some restraint

It is entirely fine to surrender and capitulate to our number one low-quality nourishments that at last fulfill our taste buds now and again. Make a point to record your desires in your food diary. I like to advise individuals to eat for fuel 90% of the time and eat for no particular reason 10%!

Try not to stop

Try not to let an intermittent mistake diversion you from adhering to your objective of turning into a better form of yourself. We are on the whole human and commit errors.

Try not to get all made up for a lost time in eating something undesirable and ruin your day as a result of it. You have the control to transform that once unfortunate day into an exceptionally solid one.

Let carbs battle for you

Against carb, perspectives are fiercely obsolete. Exploration has shown how carbs that are loaded with safe starches can assist you with feeling more fulfilled and advance by and large satiety. It enjoys energy to reprieve down these starches and causes a lessening in insulin spikes contrasted with "terrible carbs."

In all honesty, carbs are fundamental for the weight reduction game. On the off chance that you eat more sound carbs and stay away from the prepared ones, you are giving your body the fuel source it needs and likes, which furnishes you with a definitive mental fulfillment you need to continue to push forward.

Get thankful

At the point when you are starving, and at home alone, it very well may be enticing to snatch that sack of scaled-down doughnuts to nom on as opposed to picking a piece of natural product. Before you settle on s nibble, pause for a minute to stop and appreciate.

Contemplate over the fact that it is so difficult to develop products to eat, the amount you appreciate the common deliciousness of gnawing into an orange or strolling to the ranchers market. Would you be able to say any of these things regarding that sack of little doughnuts you were going to eat up?

Appreciation is one of those off-key things that can at last assistance you in your weight reduction and wellness venture. You are requiring one moment to discover the food sources that bring your sustenance, which is much harder to stop by with prepared eats. This aids in the choice interaction of settling on insightful decisions.

Try not to fear these food sources

Despite many's opinions and what you have perused consistently, the accompanying food sources at incredible on the off chance that you are taking a stab at a better waistline!

Grain and milk: While there are numerous oats out there that are loaded with abundance sugars with scarcely any health benefit, there are numerous others that have 2 ½ grams of fiber per serving. Eat these sorts with 8 ounces of entire milk to feel fulfilled in the first part of the day. Pick oats that have 10 grams or less of sugar per serving. If you are craving extra pleasantness, eat a piece of natural product!

Greek yogurt: Opt for entire milk Greek yogurt, and you will get a sound wellspring of fat that satisfies you! Eating high-fat dairy things can help in bringing down the danger of getting overweight by 8%.

Dried natural products: While numerous individuals believe that dried organic product is as terrible for you as sticky confections are, this is false. While you ought to never indulge dried natural product, these are not loaded with added sugars and is denser in calories than the crude natural product. Stacked with nutrients and fiber, it can make an extraordinary nibble with some restraint.

White potatoes: Known for their high carb content, numerous individuals make an honest effort to keep away from white potatoes. However, it isn't their carb content however much it is the structures we eat them in. From potato chips to fries showered with margarine, it is no big surprise these subterranean veggies have gotten negative criticism. Potatoes, when not canvassed in handled things, are loaded with potassium, loaded with nutrients, and are moderately low in carbohydrate level. They are acceptable carbs and increment in general satiety.

Try not to drive food varieties you disdain on yourself

Try not to feel awful on the off chance that you are not with your companions and colleagues on bouncing on the most current and most recent eating routine prevailing fashions. This doesn't mean you are off-kilter. If there are sure food sources you don't care for and appreciate, don't drive yourself to eat them.

This will just reroute you from adhering to your wellbeing objectives. It will leave you more unsatisfied than previously, and you will feel less supported.

What is an Air Fryer?

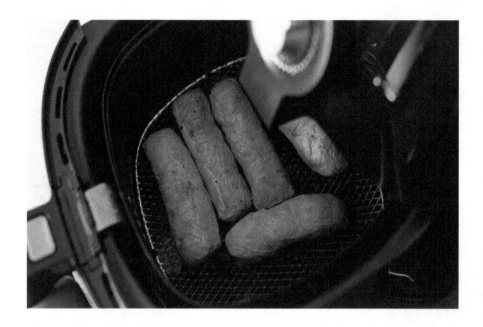

The air fryer is a moderately new kitchen apparatus used to broil food varieties with a little oil. An air fryer is the immediate partner of the conventional griddle, stove, and multi-cooker. With an air fryer, you utilize hot air as opposed to fricasseeing oil to cook dishes. With an air fryer, you can heat, meal, barbecue, and fry. You just need to utilize a little oil for preparing, broiling, cooking, and barbecuing. The air fryer warms the air to a temperature of around 400 degrees Fahrenheit. The hot air continually courses through the skillet, empowering you to cook dishes uniformly in general. This cooks all sides similarly and makes a firm covering.

Function Keys

Catch/Play/Pause Button

This Play/Pause button permits you to stop during the center of the cooking so you can shake the air fryer container or flip the food to guarantee it cooks equitably.

-/+ Button/Minus/Plus Button

This catch is utilized to change the time or temperature.

Keep Warm

This capacity keeps your food warm for 30 minutes.

Food Presets

This catch enables you to prepare food without re-thinking. The time and temperature are as of now set, so new clients discover this setting valuable.

Meal or Broil

You can dish or cook with this setting. When utilizing a traditional broiler, you need to brown the meat before cooking. You can skirt this progression when cooking with an air fryer.

Dry out

This setting prepares and dries food at a low temperature for a couple of hours. With this choice, you can make your hamburger jerky or dried natural product.

Highlights of Your Air Fryer

Versatile: The cooking gadget is convenient. The air fryer is intended to be effortlessly moved from your kitchen stockpiling cupboard to the ledge or somewhere else

Programmed temperature control: You get prepared food each time with an air fryer.

Advanced touch screen: You don't need to acquire convoluted cooking abilities, straightforwardness is inbuilt with an air fryer. With a couple of taps on the touch board's screen, you can cook an assortment of food sources.

Clock and bell: No compelling reason to stress over overcooking your food. The clock and signal will tell you when your food is prepared.

Advantages of an Air Fryer

Lessens fat substance: One reason air fryers are superior to profound fryers is the way that they help cut down on fat. At the point when you profound fry your dinners, the fat substance in your food is exceptionally high since it requires inundating your food in oil. In any case, air fryers permit you to broil your food with little oil. This assists with diminishing the fat substance in your supper.

Assists you with getting in shape: Air fryers are truly useful for weight reduction. Besides bringing down the fat substance in your feast, air fryers additionally assist you with lessening your calorie admission. The air fryer requires next to no oil to make your food fresh and crunchy, in this way diminishing your calorie consumption. At the point when profound fricasseeing food in oil, we add numerous calories, so perhaps the most appealing advantage of an air fryer is the decrease of these additional calories.

Brings down your utilization of destructive mixtures: Deep singed food sources contain a synthetic called acrylamide content. This compound is scarcely at any point present in air-seared suppers.

A lot more grounded than broiled food varieties: If you want to eat good suppers, join the number of individuals who have made air-fryer dinners their way of life.

Decrease in cooking time: With the programming of temperature and time, you can handle the consistent progression of hot air and speed up the way toward preparing food. It could set aside 40% of the time utilized in an ordinary singing interaction.

Decrease of energy use: If you look at the energy utilization of the air fryer with that of a standard electric broiler, you can see utilization fluctuates by a sensibly high rate. You can save over half of the electrical energy when utilizing the fryer. For instance, the air fryer burns through about 390Wh to sear a pound of potatoes, 45% less power than an ordinary stove employments.

Setting aside cash: You utilize less oil, and you need less energy when cooking with an air fryer. So you set aside cash.

Simple to clean: The cleaning is simpler with an air fryer. The compartment where the food is put is removable, which makes it simple to wash and clean.

Saves space: You can save kitchen space when utilizing an air fryer.

Air Fryer versus Profound Fryer

Oil use: Air fryers utilize less oil, this implies utilizing an air fryer costs you less. You need to utilize significantly more oil when profound fricasseeing. Even though you can reuse the oil, most wellbeing specialists don't suggest it.

Sound cooking: Fried food varieties, for example, air singed French fries contain up to 80% less fat in contrast with pan-fried French fries.

Cleaning: Compared to a profound fryer, cleaning an air fryer is simple. You need to clean the profound fryer and the oil fume that chooses the kitchen dividers and ledge.

Security: An air fryer is protected to utilize. With a profound fryer, there is consistently a danger of mishaps.

Different utilizations: You can just sear in a profound fryer. Then again, you can cook from various perspectives in an air fryer.

Air Fryer versus Convection Oven

Less unsafe: An air fryer gives you a one-quit cooking arrangement. With stoves, you regularly should prepare food in a prospect few moments to draw out the shading and smells before placing it in the broiler.

Safe: You can open and close the air fryer without the danger of consuming yourself. A conventional broiler presents a danger of fire.

Time: You can cook quicker in an air fryer.

Cleaning: Cleaning your air fryer is simple. Then again, cleaning a stove is tedious.

Regularly Asked Questions

Q: Can I cook various food sources noticeable all around the fryer?

A: Yes, you can cook various food varieties in your air fryer. You can utilize it for cooking various kinds of food sources like meals and even treats.

Q: How much food would I be able to put inside?

A: Different air fryers will in general have various limits. To know how much food you can place in, search for the "maximum" imprint and use it as a manual for filling the bin.

Q: Can I add fixings during the cooking interaction?

A: Yes, you can. Simply open the air fryer and add fixings. There is no compelling reason to change the interior temperature as it will balance out once you close the air fryer chamber.

Q: Can I put aluminum or preparing paper at the lower part of the air fryer?

A: Yes, you can utilize both to line the foundation of the air fryer. In any case, ensure that you punch holes so the hot air can go through the material and permit the food to prepare.

Q: Do I have to preheat?

A: Preheating the air fryer can diminish the cooking time. In any case, on the off chance that you neglected to preheat, it is still OK. To preheat the air fryer, just set it to the cooking temperature and set the clock for 5 minutes. When the clock kills, place your food in the crate and keep cooking.

Tips for the Perfect Air Fry

Discover a spot in your kitchen where it will consistently be not difficult to get to the air fryer, to the point that you need to open the cooking compartment and add your fixings.

Various plans require various temperatures to guarantee that the food is prepared appropriately. Follow the formula as accurately as conceivable to guarantee that your food tastes flavorful.

Aluminum foil assists with cleaning and is frequently used to add much more continuous control to the cooking interaction for the fixings.

Add a scramble of water when cooking greasy food sources. You will see a little cabinet at the lower part of your air fryer. This is the place where you can add a sprinkle of water when you are cooking food varieties that are high in fat. If the fat turns out to be excessively hot and dribbles to the base for a long time, it can in some cases begin to smoke. Adding vegetables forestalls smoke. In any case, on the off chance that you are just cooking meat, it is a smart thought to add water to keep the terrible smoke from rising.

Try not to pack the air fryer's cooking bushel with an excessive number of fixings. Ensure that the fixings are all at one level, particularly on the off chance that you are getting ready meat.

Flip food varieties part of the way through the cooking time if you need the two sides of your food to have a firm covering.

Try not to stress over opening the air fryer mid-cycle. In contrast to other cooking strategies, the air fryer doesn't lose heat power on the off chance that you open it trying to cook. When you close the top once more, the gadget will return to cooking temperature and keep on preparing the food.

There is a container at the lower part of the air fryer to gather oil. On the off chance that you take out both the cooking bin and the base container simultaneously and you tip them over, the oil from the base will be moved onto your plate alongside food. Thus, eliminate the base crate before serving the food. Clean the air fryer after each utilization. Extra food particles can transform into shape, create microbes, and cause terrible eventual outcomes. To stay away from this, clean the air fryer after each utilization.

When you clean the air fryer, amass everything. The air fryer will dry itself in a couple of moments.

Here is a portion of the cooking strategies that you can use with this machine:

Fry: You can keep away from oil when cooking, yet a modest quantity adds crunch and flavor to your food.

Broil: You can create excellent simmered food noticeable all around fryer
Bake: You can prepare bread, treats, and baked goods.

Flame broil: You can successfully barbecue your food, no wreck.

To begin cooking, you simply need to splash the fryer container with some cooking shower or put in a little cooking oil, add the fixings, and change the temperature and time.

Bit by bit Air Frying

Air fryers work on Rapid Air Technology. The cooking office of the air fryer discharges heat from a warming component that is near the food. The exhaust fan that is available over the cooking chamber helps in the essential wind stream from the underside. For cooking utilizing an air fryer, here are a few stages that you need to follow:

Get ready Fried Foods:

Spot the air fryer on a level and heatproof kitchen top.

Set up the food varieties.

Oil the container with a little oil and add somewhat more to the food to abstain from staying.

On the off chance that the food is marinated, wipe it off delicately to forestall splattering and abundance smoke.

Use aluminum foil for simple cleaning.

Before Cooking:

Preheat the air fryer for 3 minutes before cooking.

Abstain from congestion and leave adequate room for air course.

During Cooking time:

Add water into the air fryer cabinet to forestall unreasonable smoke and warmth Shake the crate or flip the nourishment for cooking at the midway imprint.

After Cooking:

Eliminate the bushel from the cabinet before taking out the food.

The juices noticeable all around the fryer cabinet can be utilized to make delightful marinades and sauces

Unplug, cool, and afterward clean both the crate and cabinet after use

Investigating

Food not preparing impeccably: Follow the formula precisely. Check whether you have packed the fixings. This is the principal motivation behind why food probably won't cook equitably in an air fryer.

White smoke: White smoke is generally the aftereffect of oil, so ensure that you have added some water to the base cabinet to keep the oil from overheating.

Dark smoke: Black smoke is ordinarily because of consumed food. You need to clean the air fryer after each utilization. Assuming you don't, the excess food particles are scorched when you utilize the apparatus once more. Turn the machine off and cool it. At that point check it for consumed food.

The apparatus will not stop: The aficionado of the air fryer works fast and needs an ideal opportunity to stop. Try not to stress, it will stop soon.

Cleaning Your Air Fryer

Unplug the machine and let it cool down.

Wipe the outside with a clammy fabric.

Wash the bin, plate, and dish with high temp water and cleanser. You can likewise utilize a dishwasher to wash these parts.

Clean within the air fryer with a soggy fabric or wipe.

Clean any food that is adhered to the warming component.

Dry the parts and collect the air fryer.

Tips:

Utilize clammy materials to eliminate stuck-on food. Try not to utilize utensils to abstain from scratching the non-stick covering.

On the off chance that the stuck-on food has solidified onto the bushel or dish, absorb them hot sudsy water before attempting to eliminate them.

Security Tips

Try not to purchase a modest, inferior quality air fryer.

Try not to put it on a lopsided surface.

Try not to pack the container.

Try not to leave the machine unattended.

Peruse the air fryer manual before utilizing it.

Clean the machine after each utilization.

Try not to wash the electrical parts.

Utilize the perfect measure of oil. Your air fryer needs just a little oil, so don't utilize extra.

Oil the air fryer craze. It will keep food from stalling out and forestall possible consuming and smoking.

Dry your hands before contacting the air fryer.

Ensure extras are air fryer safe.

Shake the crate or flip the food during the center of the cooking to guarantee in any event, cooking.

If your air fryer needs fixing, look for proficient help.

Breakfast Recipes

Cushioned Cheesy Omelet

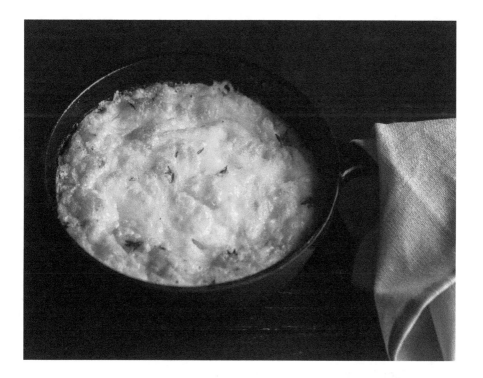

- Planning Time: 10 minutes

  Cooking time: 15 minutes

  Servings: 2

  Ingredients:

4 eggs

1 huge onion, cut

1/8 cup cheddar, ground

1/8 cup mozzarella cheddar, ground

Cooking splash

¼ teaspoon soy sauce

Newly ground dark pepper, to taste

- Directions:

Preheat the Air fryer to 360 o F and oil a container with a cooking splash.

Whisk together eggs, soy sauce, and dark pepper in a bowl.

Spot onions in the container and cook for around 10 minutes.

Pour the egg blend over onion cuts and top equally with cheddar.

Cook for around 5 additional minutes and serve.

Calories: 216, Fat: 13.8g, Carbohydrates: 7.9g, Sugar: 3.9g, Protein: 15.5g, Sodium: 251mg

Crust-Less Quiche

Planning Time: 5 minutes

Cooking time: 30 minutes

Servings: 2

- **Ingredients:**

  4 eggs

  ¼ cup onion, cleaved

  ½ cup tomatoes, cleaved

  ½ cup milk

  1 cup Gouda cheddar, destroyed

  Salt, to taste

- **Directions:**

  Preheat the Air fryer to 340 o F and oil 2 ramekins gently.

  Combine as one every one of the fixings in a ramekin until very much joined.

  Spot in the Air fryer and cook for around 30 minutes.

  Dish out and serve.

Calories: 348, Fat: 23.8g, Carbohydrates: 7.9g, Sugar: 6.3g, Protein: 26.1g, Sodium: 642mg

Chorizo Risotto

Servings: 4

Cooking Time: 1 Hour 20 Minutes

Ingredients:

- ¼ cup milk

- ½ cup flour

- 4 oz. breadcrumbs

- 4 oz. chorizo, finely cut

- 1 serving mushroom risotto rice

- 1 egg

- Ocean salt to taste

Direction:

- In a bowl, consolidate the mushroom risotto rice with the risotto and salt prior to refrigerating to cool.

- Set your Air Fryer at 390°F and leave to warm for 5 minutes.

- Utilize your hands to shape 2 tablespoonfuls of risotto into a rice ball. Rehash until you have spent all the risotto. Roll each ball in the flour.

- Break the egg into a bowl and blend in with the milk utilizing a whisk. Coat each rice ball in the egg-milk blend, and afterward in breadcrumbs.

- Space the rice balls out in the preparing dish of the Air Fryer. Prepare for 20 minutes, guaranteeing they build up a firm brilliant earthy colored covering.

- Serve warm with a side of new vegetables and salad whenever wanted.

Egg Yolks With Squid

Servings:4

Cooking Time: 20 Minutes

Ingredients:

- ½ cup self-rising flour

- 14 ounces squid bloom, cleaned and pat dried

- Salt and newly ground dark pepper

- 1 tablespoon olive oil

- 2 tablespoons margarine

- 2 green chilies, cultivated and slashed

- 2 curry leaves stalks

- 4 crude salted egg yolks

- ½ cup chicken stock

- 2 tablespoons vanished milk

- 1 tablespoon sugar

Directions:

- Set the temperature of Air Fryer to 355 degrees F. Oil an Air Fryer skillet.

- In a shallow dish, add the flour.

- Sprinkle the squid bloom equitably with salt and dark pepper.

- Coat the squid equitably with flour and afterward shake off any overabundance flour.

- Spot the squid into the readied skillet in a solitary layer.

- Air Fry for around 9 minutes.

- Eliminate from the Air Fryer and put away

- Presently, heat the oil and spread in a skillet over medium warmth and sauté the chilies and curry leaves for around 3 minutes.

- Add the egg yolks and cook for around 1 moment, blending persistently.

- Steadily, add the chicken stock and cook for around 3-5 minutes, mixing constantly.

- Include the milk and sugar and blend until all around consolidated.

- Add the seared squid and throw to cover well.

- Serve hot.

Parsnip Hash Browns

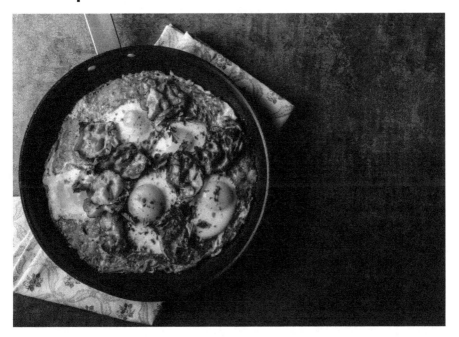

Servings: 2

Cooking Time:
20 Minutes

Ingredients:

- 3 eggs, beaten

- ½ tsp garlic powder

- ¼ tsp nutmeg

- 1 tbsp olive oil

- 1 cup flour

- Salt and pepper, to taste

Directions:

- Heat olive oil in the air fryer at 390 F. In a bowl, combine flour, eggs, parsnip, nutmeg, and garlic powder. Season with salt and pepper. Form patties out of the mixture. Arrange in the air fryer and cook for minutes.

Very Berry Breakfast Puffs

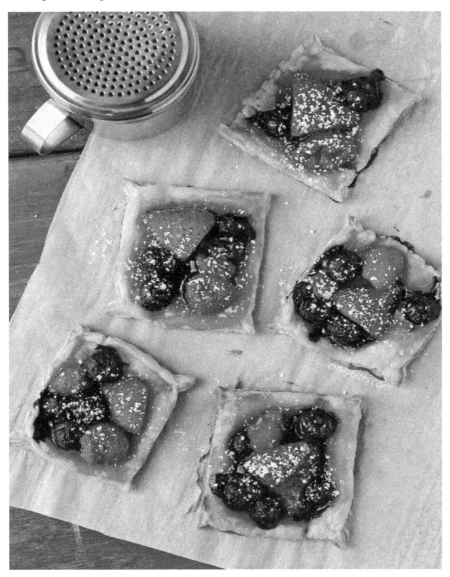

Servings:3

Cooking Time: 20
 Minutes

Ingredients:

- 2 tbsp mashed strawberries

- 2 tbsp mashed raspberries

- ¼ tsp vanilla extract

- 2 cups cream cheese

- 1 tbsp honey

Directions:

- Preheat the air fryer to 375 F. Divide the cream cheese between the dough sheets and spread it evenly. In a small bowl, combine the berries, honey and vanilla.

- Divide the mixture between the pastry sheets. Pinch the ends of the sheets, to form puff. Place the puffs on a lined baking dish. Place the dish in the air fryer and cook for 15 minutes.

Milky Scrambled Eggs

Preparation Time: 10 minutes

Cooking time: 9 minutes

Servings: 2

Ingredients:

- ¾ cup milk

- 4 eggs

- 8 grape tomatoes, halved

- ½ cup Parmesan cheese, grated

- 1 tablespoon butter

- Salt and black pepper, to taste

Directions:

- Preheat the Air fryer to 360 o F and grease an Air fryer pan with butter.

- Whisk together eggs with milk, salt and black pepper in a bowl.

- Transfer the egg mixture into the prepared pan and place in the Air fryer.

- Cook for about 6 minutes and stir in the grape tomatoes and cheese.

- Cook for about 3 minutes and serve warm.

Nutrition:

Calories: 351, Fat: 22g, Carbohydrates: 25.2g, Sugar: 17.7g, Protein: 26.4g, Sodium: 422mg

Toasties and Sausage in Egg Pond

Preparation Time: 10 minutes

Cooking time: 22 minutes

Servings: 2

Ingredients:

- 3 eggs

- 2 cooked sausages, sliced

- 1 bread slice, cut into sticks

- 1/8 cup mozzarella cheese, grated

- 1/8 cup Parmesan cheese, grated ¼ cup cream

Directions:

- Preheat the Air fryer to 365 o F and grease 2 ramekins lightly.

- Whisk together eggs with cream in a bowl and place in the ramekins.

- Stir in the bread and sausage slices in the egg mixture and top with cheese.

- Transfer the ramekins in the Air fryer basket and cook for about 22 minutes. Dish out and serve warm.

Nutrition:

Calories: 261, Fat: 18.8g, Carbohydrates: 4.2g, Sugar: 1.3g, Protein: 18.3g, Sodium: 428mg

Banana Bread

Preparation Time: 10 minutes

Cooking time: 20 minutes

Servings: 8

Ingredients:

- 1 1/3 cups flour

- 1 teaspoon baking soda

- 1 teaspoon baking powder

- ½ cup milk

- 3 bananas, peeled and sliced

- 2/3 cup sugar

- 1 teaspoon ground cinnamon

- 1 teaspoon salt ½ cup olive oil

Directions:

- Preheat the Air fryer to 330 o F and grease a loaf pan.

- Mix together all the dry ingredients with the wet ingredients to form a dough.

- Place the dough into the prepared loaf pan and transfer into an air fryer basket.

- Cook for about 20 minutes and remove from air fryer.

- Cut the bread into desired size slices and serve warm.

Nutrition: Calories: 295, Fat: 13.3g, Carbohydrates: 44g, Sugar: 22.8g, Protein: 3.1g, Sodium: 458mg

Flavorful Bacon Cups

Preparation Time: 10 minutes

Cooking time: 15 minutes

Servings: 6

Ingredients:

- 6 bacon slices

- 6 bread slices

- 1 scallion, chopped

- 3 tablespoons green bell pepper, seeded and chopped

- 6 eggs

- 2 tablespoons low-fat mayonnaise

Directions:

- Preheat the Air fryer to 375 o F and grease 6 cups muffin tin with cooking spray.

- Place each bacon slice in a prepared muffin cup.

- Cut the bread slices with round cookie cutter and place over the bacon slices.

- Top with bell pepper, scallion and mayonnaise evenly and crack 1 egg in each muffin cup.

- Place in the Air fryer and cook for about 15 minutes.

- Dish out and serve warm.

Nutrition:

Calories: 260, Fat: 18g, Carbohydrates: 6.9g, Sugar: 1.03g, Protein: 16.7g, Sodium: 805mg

Lunch Recipes

Yogurt Garlic Chicken

Preparation Time: 30 min

Cooking time: 60 min

Servings: 6

Ingredients:

- Pita bread rounds, halved (6 pieces)

- English cucumber, sliced thinly, w/ each slice halved (1 cup)

- Olive oil (3 tablespoons)

- Black pepper, freshly ground (1/2 teaspoon)

- Chicken thighs, skinless, boneless (20 ounces)

- Bell pepper, red, sliced into half-inch portions (1 piece)

- Garlic cloves, chopped finely (4 pieces)

- Cumin, ground (1/2 teaspoon)

- Red onion, medium, sliced into half-inch wedges (1 piece)

- Yogurt, plain, fat free (1/2 cup)

- Lemon juice (2 tablespoons)

- Salt (1 ½ teaspoons)

- Red pepper flakes, crushed (1/2 teaspoon)

- Allspice, ground (1/2 teaspoon)

- Bell pepper, yellow, sliced into half-inch portions (1 piece)

- Yogurt sauce

- Olive oil (2 tablespoons)

- Salt (1/4 teaspoon)

- Parsley, flat leaf, chopped finely (1 tablespoon)

- Yogurt, plain, fat free (1 cup)

- Lemon juice, fresh (1 tablespoon)

- Garlic clove, chopped finely (1 piece)

Directions:

- Mix the yogurt (1/2 cup), garlic cloves (4 pieces), olive oil (1 tablespoon), salt (1 teaspoon), lemon juice (2 tablespoons), pepper (1/4 teaspoon), allspice, cumin, and pepper flakes. Stir in the chicken and coat well. Cover and marinate in the fridge for two hours.

- Preheat the air fryer at 400 degrees Fahrenheit.

- Grease a rimmed baking sheet (18x13-inch) with cooking spray. Toss the bell peppers and onion with remaining olive oil (2 tablespoons), pepper (1/4 teaspoon), and salt (1/2 teaspoon).

- Arrange veggies on the baking sheet's left side and the marinated chicken thighs (drain first) on the right side. Cook in the air fryer for twenty-five to thirty minutes.

- Mix the yogurt sauce ingredients.

- Slice air-fried chicken into half-inch strips.

- Top each pita round with chicken strips, roasted veggies, cucumbers, and yogurt sauce.

Nutrition: Calories 380 Fat 15.0 g Protein 26.0 g Carbohydrates 34.0 g

Lemony Parmesan Salmon

Preparation Time: 10 min

Cooking time: 25 min

Servings: 4

Ingredients:

- Butter, melted (2 tablespoons)

- Green onions, sliced thinly (2 tablespoons)

- Breadcrumbs, white, fresh (3/4 cup)

- Thyme leaves, dried (1/4 teaspoon)

- Salmon fillet, 1 ¼-pound (1 piece)

- Salt (1/4 teaspoon)

- Parmesan cheese, grated (1/4 cup) Lemon peel, grated (2 teaspoons)

Directions:

- Preheat the air fryer at 350 degrees Fahrenheit.

- Mist cooking spray onto a baking pan (shallow). Fill with pat-dried salmon. Brush salmon with butter (1 tablespoon) before sprinkling with salt.

- Combine the breadcrumbs with onions, thyme, lemon peel, cheese, and remaining butter (1 tablespoon).

- Cover salmon with the breadcrumb mixture. Air-fry for fifteen to twentyfive minutes.

Nutrition: Calories 290 Fat 16.0 g Protein 33.0 g Carbohydrates 4.0 g

Easiest Tuna Cobbler Ever

Preparation time: 15 min Cooking time: 25 min

Servings: 4

Ingredients:

- Water, cold (1/3 cup)

- Tuna, canned, drained (10 ounces)

- Sweet pickle relish (2 tablespoons)

- Mixed vegetables, frozen (1 ½ cups)

- Soup, cream of chicken, condensed (10 ¾ ounces)

- Pimientos, sliced, drained (2 ounces)

- Lemon juice (1 teaspoon)

- Paprika

Directions:

- Preheat the air fryer at 375 degrees Fahrenheit.

- Mist cooking spray into a round casserole (1 ½ quarts).

- Mix the frozen vegetables with milk, soup, lemon juice, relish, pimientos, and tuna in a saucepan. Cook for six to eight minutes over medium heat. Fill the casserole with the tuna mixture.

- Mix the biscuit mix with cold water to form a soft dough. Beat for half a minute before dropping by four spoonfuls into the casserole. Dust the dish with paprika before air-frying for twenty to twenty-five minutes.

Nutrition: Calories 320 Fat 11.0 g Protein 28.0 g Carbohydrates 31.0 g

Homemade Pork Buns

Preparation time: 20 min

Cooking time: 25 min

Servings: 8

Ingredients:

- Green onions, sliced thinly (3 pieces)

- Egg, beaten (1 piece)

- Pulled pork, diced, w/ barbecue sauce (1 cup)

- Buttermilk biscuits, refrigerated (16 1/3 ounces) Soy sauce (1 teaspoon)

Directions:

- Preheat the air fryer at 325 degrees Fahrenheit.

- Use parchment paper to line your baking sheet.

- Combine pork with green onions.

- Separate and press the dough to form 8 four-inch rounds.

- Fill each biscuit round's center with two tablespoons of pork mixture. Cover with the dough edges and seal by pinching. Arrange the buns on the sheet and brush with a mixture of soy sauce and egg.

- Cook in the air fryer for twenty to twenty-five minutes.

Nutrition: Calories 240 Fat 9.0 g Protein 8.0 g Carbohydrates 29.0 g

Chili Bell Peppers Stew

Servings: 4

CookingTime: 15Minutes

Ingredients:

2 red bell peppers, cut into wedges

2 green bell peppers, cut into wedges

2 yellow bell peppers, cut into wedges

½ cup keto tomato sauce

1 tablespoon chili powder

2 teaspoons cumin, ground

¼ teaspoon sweet paprika

Salt and black pepper to the taste

Directions:

In a pan that fits your air fryer, mix all the ingredients, toss, introduce the pan in the machine and cook at 370 degrees F for minutes. Divide into bowls and serve for lunch.

Grilled Ham & Cheese

Servings: 2

Cooking Time: 30 Minutes

Ingredients:

>   3l ow-carb buns
>
>   4 slices medium-cut deli ham
>
>   1 tbsp salted butter
>
>   1 oz. flour
>
>   3 slices cheddar cheese
>
>   3 slices muenster cheese

Directions:

>   Bread:
>
>   Preheat your fryer to 350°F/175°C.
>
>   Mix the flour, salt and baking powder in a bowl. Put to the side.
>
>   Add in the butter and coconut oil to a skillet.
>
>   Melt for 20 seconds and pour into another bowl.
>
>   In this bowl, mix in the dough.

Scramble two eggs. Add to the dough.

Add ½ tablespoon of coconut flour to thicken, and place evenly into a cupcake tray. Fill about ¾ inch.

Bake for 20 minutes until browned.

Allow to cool for 15 minutes and cut each in half for the buns.

Sandwich:

Fry the deli meat in a skillet on a high heat.

Put the ham and cheese between the buns.

Heat the butter on medium high.

When brown, turn to low and add the dough to pan.

Press down with a weight until you smell burning, then flip to crisp both sides.

Enjoy!

Thyme Green Beans

Servings: 6

Cooking Time: 20 Minutes

Ingredients:

> 1 pound green beans, trimmed and halved
>
> 2 eggplants, cubed
>
> 1 cup veggie stock
>
> 1 tablespoon olive oil
>
> 1 red chili pepper
>
> 1 red bell pepper, chopped
>
> ½ teaspoon thyme, dried
>
> Salt and black pepper to the taste

Directions:

> In a pan that fits your air fryer, mix all the ingredients, toss, introduce the pan in the machine and cook at 350 degrees F for 20 minutes. Divide into bowls and serve for lunch.

Rosemary Lamb

Servings: 4

Cooking Time: 30 Minutes

Ingredients:

- tablespoon olive oil

- garlic clove, minced

- 1 tablespoon rosemary, chopped

- ¼ cup keto tomato sauce

- 1 cup baby spinach

- 1 and ½ pounds lamb, cubed

- Salt and black pepper to the taste

Directions:

- Heat up a pan that fits the air fryer with the oil over medium heat, add the lamb and garlic and brown for 5 minutes. Add the rest of the ingredients except the spinach, introduce the pan in the fryer and cook at 390 degrees F for minutes, shaking the machine halfway. Add the spinach, cook for 10 minutes more, divide between plates and serve for lunch.

Meat Bake

Servings: 4

Cooking Time: 30 Minutes

Ingredients:

- 1 pound lean beef, cubed
- 1 pound pork stew meat, cubed
- tablespoon spring onions, chopped
- tablespoons keto tomato sauce
- A drizzle of olive oil
- A pinch of salt and black pepper
- ¼ teaspoon sweet paprika

Directions:

- Heat up a pan that fits the air fryer with the oil over medium-high heat, add the pork and beef meat and brown for 5 minutes. Add the remaining ingredients, toss, introduce the pan in the air fryer and cook at 390 degrees F for 25 minutes. Divide the mix between plates and serve for lunch with a side salad.

Mouthwatering Tuna Melts

Cooking time: 20 min

Servings: 8

Ingredients:

- Salt (1/8 teaspoon)

- Onion, chopped (1/3 cup)

- Biscuits, refrigerated, flaky layers (16 1/3 ounces)

- Tuna, water packed, drained (10 ounces)

- Mayonnaise (1/3 cup) Pepper (1/8 teaspoon)
- Cheddar cheese, shredded (4 ounces)

- Tomato, chopped

- Sour cream

- Lettuce, shredded

Directions:

- Preheat the air fryer at 325 degrees Fahrenheit.

- Mist cooking spray onto a cookie sheet.

- Mix tuna with mayonnaise, pepper, salt, and onion.

- Separate dough so you have 8 biscuits; press each into 5-inch rounds.

- Arrange 4 biscuit rounds on the sheet. Fill at the center with tuna mixture before topping with cheese. Cover with the remaining biscuit rounds and press to seal.

- Air-fry for fifteen to twenty minutes. Slice each sandwich into halves. Serve each piece topped with lettuce, tomato, and sour cream.

Nutrition: Calories 320 Fat 18.0 g Protein 14.0 g Carbohydrates 27.0 g

Poultry Recipes

Creamy Coconut Chicken

Preparation time: 2 hours Cooking time:
25 minutes Servings: 4

Ingredients:

- 4 big chicken legs

- 4 teaspoons turmeric powder

- 2 tablespoons ginger, grated

- Salt and black pepper to the taste

- 4 tablespoons coconut cream

Directions:

- In a bowl, mix cream with turmeric, ginger, salt and pepper, whisk, add chicken pieces, toss them well and leave aside for 2 hours.

- Transfer chicken to your preheated air fryer, cook at 370 degrees F for 25 minutes, divide among plates and serve with a side salad.

Enjoy!

Nutrition: calories 300, fat 4, fiber 12, carbs 22, protein 20

Chinese Chicken Wings

Preparation time: 2 hours

Cooking time: 15 minutes

Servings: 6

Ingredients:

- 16 chicken wings

- 2 tablespoons honey

- tablespoons soy sauce

- Salt and black pepper to the taste

- ¼ teaspoon white pepper

- tablespoons lime juice

Directions:

- In a bowl, mix honey with soy sauce, salt, black and white pepper and lime juice, whisk well, add chicken pieces, toss to coat and keep in the fridge for 2 hours.

- Transfer chicken to your air fryer, cook at 370 degrees F for 6 minutes on each side, increase heat to 400 degrees F and cook for 3 minutes more.

- Serve hot.

Enjoy!

Nutrition: calories 372, fat 9, fiber 10, carbs 37, protein 24

Herbed Chicken

Preparation time: 30 minutes

Cooking time: 40 minutes

Servings: 4

Ingredients:

- 1 whole chicken

- Salt and black pepper to the taste

- 1 teaspoon garlic powder 1 teaspoon onion powder

- ½ teaspoon thyme, dried

- 1 teaspoon rosemary, dried

- tablespoon lemon juice

- tablespoons olive oil

Directions:

- Use pepper and salt to season the chicken, mix with thyme, rosemary, garlic powder and onion powder, rub with lemon juice and olive oil and leave aside for 30 minutes.

- Put chicken in your air fryer and cook at 360 degrees F for 20 minutes on each side.

- Leave chicken aside to cool down, carve and serve.

Enjoy!

Nutrition: calories 390, fat 10, fiber 5, carbs 22, protein 20

Chicken Parmesan

Preparation time:10minutes

Cooking time: 15minutes

Servings: 4

Ingredients:

- 2 cups panko bread crumbs

- ¼ cup parmesan, grated

- ½ teaspoon garlic powder

- 2 cups white flour

- 1 egg, whisked

- 1 and ½ pounds chicken cutlets, skinless and boneless

- Salt and black pepper to the taste

- cup mozzarella, grated

- cups tomato sauce

- tablespoons basil, chopped

Directions:

- In a bowl, mix panko with parmesan and garlic powder and stir.

- Put flour in a second bowl and the egg in a third.

- Season chicken with salt and pepper, dip in flour, then in egg mix and in panko.

- Put chicken pieces in your air fryer and cook them at 360 degrees F for 3 minutes on each side.

- Transfer chicken to a baking dish that fits your air fryer, add tomato sauce and top with mozzarella, introduce in your air fryer and cook at 375 degrees F for 7 minutes.

- Divide among plates, sprinkle basil on top and serve.

Enjoy!

Nutrition: calories 304, fat 12, fiber 11, carbs 22, protein 15

Mexican Chicken

Preparation time: 10 minutes

Cooking time: 20 minutes

Servings: 4

Ingredients:

- 16 ounces salsa verde

- 1 tablespoon olive oil

- Salt and black pepper to the taste

- 1 pound chicken breast, boneless and skinless

- 1 and ½ cup Monterey Jack cheese, grated

- ¼ cup cilantro, chopped 1 teaspoon garlic powder

Directions:

- Pour salsa verde in a baking dish that fits your air fryer, season chicken with salt, pepper, garlic powder, brush with olive oil and place it over your salsa verde. put in your air fryer and boil at 380 degrees F for 20 minutes.

- Sprinkle cheese on top and cook for 2 minutes more.

- Divide among plates and serve hot.

Enjoy!

Nutrition: calories 340, fat 18, fiber 14, carbs 32, protein 18

Creamy Chicken, Rice and Peas

Preparation time: 10 minutes

Cooking time: 30 minutes

Servings: 4

Ingredients:

- 1 pound chicken breasts, skinless, boneless and cut into quarters

- 1 cup white rice, already cooked

- Salt and black pepper to the taste

- 1 tablespoon olive oil

- 3 garlic cloves, minced

- 1 yellow onion, chopped

- ½ cup white wine

- ¼ cup heavy cream

- cup chicken stock

- ¼ cup parsley, chopped

- cups peas, frozen

- 1 and ½ cups parmesan, grated

Directions:

- Season chicken breasts with salt and pepper, drizzle half of the oil over them, rub well, put in your air fryer's basket and cook them at 360 degrees F for 6 minutes.

- Warm the pot with the remaining oil over medium high heat, add garlic, onion, wine, stock, salt, pepper and heavy cream, stir, bring to a simmer and cook for 9 minutes.

- Transfer chicken breasts to a heat proof dish that fits your air fryer, add peas, rice and cream mix over them, toss, sprinkle parmesan and parsley all over, place in your air fryer and cook at 420 degrees F for 10 minutes.

- Divide among plates and serve hot.

Enjoy!

Nutrition: calories 313, fat 12, fiber 14, carbs 27, protein 44

Prune-stuffed Turkey Tenderloins

Servings:4

Cooking Time:1Hour

Ingredients:

- 3/4 cup prunes, pitted and chopped

- 1/2 teaspoon dried marjoram

- sprig thyme, leaves only, crushed

- tablespoons fresh coriander, minced

- 1/4 teaspoon ground allspice

- 1/2 cup softened butter

- ½ pounds turkey tenderloins

- tablespoons dry white wine

Directions:

- In a mixing bowl, thoroughly combine the first 6 ingredients; stir with a spoon until everything is well shared.

- Cut the "pockets" into the sides of the turkey tenderloins. Stuff them with prepared prune mixture. Now, tie each "pocket" with a cooking twine. Sprinkle them with white wine.

- Cook the stuffed turkey in the preheated Air Fryer at 5 degrees F for 48 to 55 minutes, checking periodically.

- Afterward, remove cooking twine, cut each turkey tenderloin into

2 slices and serve immediately.

Sweet & Sour Chicken Thighs

Servings:2

Cooking Time: 20Minutes

Ingredients:

- 1 scallion, finely chopped

- 1 garlic clove, minced

- ½ tablespoon soy sauce

- ½ tablespoon rice vinegar

- teaspoon sugar

- Salt and ground black pepper, as required

- (4-ounces) skinless, boneless chicken thighs

- ½ cup corn flour

Directions:

- Mix together all the ingredients except chicken, and corn flour in a bowl.

- Add the chicken thighs and generously coat with marinade.

- Add the corn flour in another bowl.

- Remove the chicken thighs from marinade and coat with corn flour.

- Set the temperature of Air Fryer to 390 degrees F. Grease an Air Fryer basket.

- Arrange chicken thighs into the prepared Air Fryer basket, skin side down.

- Air Fry for about 10 minutes and then another 10 minutes at 355 degrees F.

- Remove from Air Fryer and transfer the chicken thighs onto a serving platter.

- Serve hot.

Oregano And Lemon Chicken Drumsticks

Servings: 4

Cooking Time: 21
Minutes

Ingredients:

- 4 chicken drumsticks, with skin, bone-in

- 1 teaspoon dried cilantro

- ½ teaspoon dried oregano

- ½ teaspoon salt

- 1 teaspoon lemon juice

- teaspoon butter, softened

- garlic cloves, diced

Directions:

- In the mixing bowl mix up dried cilantro, oregano, and salt. Then fill the chicken drumstick's skin with a cilantro mixture. Add butter and diced garlic. Sprinkle the chicken with lemon juice. Preheat the air fryer to 375F. Put the chicken drumsticks in the air fryer and cook them for 2minutes.

Paprika-cumin Rubbed Chicken Tenderloin

Servings:6

Cooking Time:25Minutes

Ingredients:

- ¼ cup coconut flour

- ¼ cup olive oil

- ½ teaspoon garlic powder

- ½ teaspoon ground cumin

- ½ teaspoon onion powder

- ½ teaspoon smoked paprika

- 1-pound chicken tenderloins Salt and pepper to taste

Directions:

- Preheat the air fryer for 5 minutes.

- Soak the chicken tenderloins in olive oil.

- Mix the rest of the ingredients and stir using your hands to combine everything.

- Place the chicken pieces in the air fryer basket.

- Cook for 2minutes at 3250F.

Fish and Seafood Recipe

Cajun Style Shrimp

Preparation time: 3 minutes

Cooking time: 10 minutes

Servings: 2

Ingredients:

- 6g of salt

- 2g smoked paprika

- 2g garlic powder

- 2g Italian seasoning

- 2g chili powder

- 1g onion powder

- 1g cayenne pepper

- 1g black pepper

- 1g dried thyme

- 454g large shrimp, peeled and unveiled

- 30 ml of olive oil Lime wedges, to serve

Directions:

- Select Preheat, in the air fryer, set the temperature to 190°C and press Start/Pause.

- Combine all seasonings in a large bowl. Set aside

- Mix the shrimp with olive oil until they are evenly coated.

- Sprinkle the dressing mixture over the shrimp and stir until well coated.

- Place the shrimp in the preheated air fryer.

- Select Shrimp set the time to 5 minutes and press Start/Pause.

- Shake the baskets in the middle of cooking.

- Serve with pieces of lime.

Nutrition:

Calories: 126, Fat: 6g, Carbohydrates: 2g, Proteins: 33g, Cholesterol: 199mg, Sodium: 231mg.

Crab Cakes

Preparation time: 10 minutes

Cooking time: 40 minutes

Servings: 2

Ingredients:

For crab cakes:

- 1 large egg, beaten
- 17g of mayonnaise
- 11g Dijon mustard
- 5 ml Worcestershire sauce
- 2g Old Bay seasoning
- 2g of salt
- A pinch of white pepper
- A pinch of cayenne
- 26g celery, finely diced
- 45g red pepper, finely diced
- 8g fresh parsley, finely chopped
- 227g of crab meat
- 28g breadcrumbs Nonstick Spray Oil

Remodeled:

- 55g of mayonnaise

- 15g capers, washed and drained

- 5g sweet pickles, chopped

- 5g red onion, finely chopped

- 8 ml of lemon juice

- 8g Dijon mustard

- Salt and pepper to taste

Directions:

- Mix the ingredients of remodeled until everything is well incorporated. Set aside

- Beat the egg, mayonnaise, mustard, Worcestershire sauce, Old Bay seasoning, salt, white pepper, cayenne pepper, celery, pepper, and parsley.

- Gently stir the crab meat in the egg mixture and stir it until well mixed.

- Sprinkle the breadcrumbs over the crab mixture and fold them gently until the breadcrumbs cover every corner.

- Shape the crab mixture into 4 cakes and chill in the fridge for 30 minutes.

- Select Preheat in the air fryer and press Start/Pause.

- Place a sheet of baking paper in the basket of the preheated air fryer. Sprinkle the crab cakes with cooking spray and place them gently on the paper.

- Cook the crab cakes at 205°C for 8 minutes until golden brown.

- Flip crab cakes during cooking.

- Serve with remodeled.

Nutrition:

Calories: 110, Fat: 6.5g, Carbohydrates: 5.5g Protein: 7, Sugar: 2g

Tuna Pie

Preparation time: 10 minutes

Cooking time: 30 minutes

Servings: 4

Ingredients:

- 2 hard-boiled eggs

- 2 tuna cans 200 ml fried tomato 1 sheet of broken dough.

Directions:

- Cut the eggs into small pieces and mix with the tuna and tomato.

- Spread the sheet of broken dough and cut into two equal squares.

- Put the mixture of tuna, eggs, and tomato on one of the squares.

- Cover with the other, join at the ends and decorate with leftover little pieces.

- Preheat the air fryer a few minutes at 1800C.

- Enter in the air fryer basket and set the timer for 15 minutes at 1800C

Nutrition:

Calories: 244, Fat: 13.67g, Carbohydrates: 21.06g, Protein: 8.72g

Sugar: 0.22g, Cholesterol: 59mg

Tuna Puff Pastry

Preparation time: 5 minutes

Cooking time: 15 minutes

Servings: 2

Ingredients:

- 2 square puff pastry dough, bought ready

- 1 egg (white and yolk separated)

- ½ cup tuna tea

- ½ cup chopped parsley tea

- ½ cup chopped tea olives Salt and pepper to taste

Directions:

- Preheat the air fryer. Set the timer of 5 minutes and the temperature to 200C.

- Mix the tuna with olives and parsley. Season to taste and set aside. Place half of the filling in each dough and fold in half. Brush with egg white and close gently. After closing, make two small cuts at the top of the air outlet. Brush with the egg yolk.

- Place in the basket of the air fryer. Set the time to 10 minutes and press the power button.

Nutrition:

Calories: 291, Fat: 16g, Carbohydrates: 26g, Protein: 8g, Sugar: 0g

Cholesterol: 0

Cajun Style Catfish

Preparation time: 3 minutes

Cooking time: 7 minutes

Servings: 2

Ingredients:

- 5g of paprika
- 3g garlic powder 2g onion powder
- 2g ground dried thyme
- 1g ground black pepper
- 1g cayenne pepper
- 1g dried basil
- 1g dried oregano
- 2 catfish fillets (6 oz) Nonstick Spray Oil

Direction:

- Preheat the air fryer for a few minutes. Set the temperature to 175°C.
- Mix all seasonings in a bowl.
- Cover the fish generously on each side with the dressing mixture. Spray each side of the fish with oil spray and place it in the preheated air fryer.

- Select Marine Food and press Start /Pause.

- Remove carefully when you finish cooking and serve on semolina.

Nutrition:

Calories: 228, Fat; 13g, Carbohydrates: 0g, Protein: 20g, Sugar: 0g

Cholesterol: 71mg

Meat Recipes

Lime Lamb Mix

Preparation time: 5 minutes

Cooking time: 30 minutes

Servings: 4

Ingredients:

- 2pounds lamb chops

- Juice of 1 lime

- Zest of 1 lime, grated

- A pinch of salt and black pepper

- 1tablespoon olive oil

- 1teaspoon sweet paprika

- 1teaspoon cumin, ground

- 1tablespoon cumin, ground

Directions:

- In the air fryer's basket, mix the lamb chops with the lime juice and the other ingredients, rub and cook at 380 degrees F for 15 minutes on each side.

- Serve with a side salad.

Nutrition: Calories 284, Fat 13, Fiber 3, Carbs 5, Protein 15

Lamb and Corn

Cooking time: 30 minutes

Servings: 4

Ingredients:

- 2pounds lamb stew meat, cubed

- 1cup corn

- 1cup spring onions, chopped

- ¼ cup beef stock

- 1tablespoon olive oil

- A pinch of salt and black pepper

- 2tablespoons rosemary, chopped

Directions:

- In the air fryer's pan, mix the lamb with the corn, spring onions and the other ingredients, toss and cook at 380 degrees F for 30 minutes.

- Divide the mix between plates and serve.

Nutrition: Calories 274, Fat 12, Fiber 3, Carbs 5, Protein 15

Herbed Beef and Squash

Preparation time: 10 minutes

Cooking time: 30 minutes

Servings: 4

Ingredients:

- 2pounds beef stew meat, cubed

- 1cup butternut squash, peeled and cubed

- 1tablespoon basil, chopped

- 1tablespoon oregano, chopped

- A pinch of salt and black pepper

- A drizzle of olive oil

- 2garlic cloves, minced

Directions:

- In the air fryer's pan, mix the beef with the squash and the other ingredients, toss and cook at 380 degrees F for 30 minutes.

- Divide between plates and serve.

Nutrition: Calories 284, Fat 13, Fiber 3, Carbs 6, Protein 14

Smoked Beef Mix

Cooking time: 20 minutes

Servings: 4

Ingredients:

- 1pound beef stew meat, roughly cubed

- 1tablespoon smoked paprika

- ½ cup beef stock

- ½ teaspoon garam masala

- 2tablespoons olive oil

- A pinch of salt and black pepper

Directions:

- In the air fryer's basket, mix the beef with the smoked paprika and the other ingredients, toss and cook at 390 degrees F for 20 minutes on each side.

- Divide between plates and serve.

Nutrition: Calories 274, Fat 12, Fiber 4, Carbs 6, Protein 17

Marjoram Pork Mix

Cooking time: 25 minutes

Servings: 4

Ingredients:

- 2pounds pork stew meat, roughly cubed

- 1tablespoon marjoram, chopped

- 1cup heavy cream

- 2tablespoons olive oil

- Salt and black pepper to the taste

- 2garlic cloves, minced

Directions:

- Heat up a pan that fits the air fryer with the oil over medium-high heat, add the meat and brown for 5 minutes

- Add the rest of the ingredients, toss, put the pan in the fryer and cook at 400 degrees F for 20 minutes more.

- Divide between plates and serve.

Nutrition: Calories 274, Fat 14, Fiber 3, Carbs 6, Protein 14

Nutmeg Lamb

Servings: 4

Ingredients:

- 1pound lamb stew meat, cubed

- 2teaspoons nutmeg, ground

- 1teaspoon coriander, ground

- 1cup heavy cream

- 2tablespoons olive oil

- 2tablespoons chives, chopped

- Salt and black pepper to the taste

Directions:

- In the air fryer's pan, mix the lamb with the nutmeg and the other ingredients, put the pan in the air fryer and cook at 380 degrees F for 30 minutes.

- Divide everything into bowls and serve.

Nutrition: Calories 287, Fat 13, Fiber 2, Carbs 6, Protein 12

Greek Beef Mix

Servings: 4

Ingredients:

- 2pounds beef stew meat, roughly cubed

- 1teaspoon coriander, ground

- 1teaspoon garam masala

- 1teaspoon cumin, ground

- A pinch of salt and black pepper

- 1cup Greek yogurt

- ½ teaspoon turmeric powder

Directions:

- In the air fryer's pan, mix the beef with the coriander and the other ingredients, toss and cook at 380 degrees F for 30 minutes.

- Divide between plates and serve.

Nutrition: Calories 283, Fat 13, Fiber 3, Carbs 6, Protein 15

Beef and Fennel

Servings: 4

Ingredients:

- 2pounds beef stew meat, cut into strips

- 2fennel bulbs, sliced

- 2tablespoons mustard

- A pinch of salt and black pepper

- 1tablespoon black peppercorns, ground

- 2tablespoons balsamic vinegar

- 2tablespoons olive oil

Directions:

- In the air fryer's pan, mix the beef with the fennel and the other ingredients.

- Put the pan in the fryer and cook at 380 degrees for 30 minutes.

- Divide everything into bowls and serve.

Nutrition: Calories 283, Fat 13, Fiber 2, Carbs 6, Protein 17

Side Dish Recipes

Easy Polenta Pie

Preparation time: 10 min

Cooking time: 55 min

Servings: 6

Ingredients:

- Egg, slightly beaten (1 piece)

- Water (2 cups)

- Monterey Jack cheese, w/ jalapeno peppers, shredded (3/4 cup)

- Cornmeal (3/4 cup)

- Salt (1/4 teaspoon)

- Chili beans, drained (15 ounces) Tortilla chips/crushed corn (1/3 cup)

Directions:

- Preheat air fryer at 350 degrees Fahrenheit.

- Mist cooking spray onto a pie plate.

- In saucepan heated on medium-high, combine water, salt, and cornmeal. Let mixture boil, then cook on medium heat for six minutes. Stir in egg and let sit for five minutes.

- Pour cornmeal mixture into pie plate and spread evenly. Air-fry for fifteen minutes and top with beans, corn chips, and cheese. Air-fry for another twenty minutes.

Nutrition: Calories 195 Fat 7.0 g Protein 10.0 g Carbohydrates 27.0 g

Bean and Rice Dish

Preparation time: 10 min

Cooking time: 1 hr 5 min

Servings: 4

Ingredients:

- Boiling water (1 ½ cups)

- Kidney beans, dark red, undrained (15 ounces)

- Marjoram leaves, dried (1/2 teaspoon)

- Cheddar cheese, shredded (1/2 cup)

- White rice, long grain, uncooked (1 cup)

- Bouillon, chicken/vegetable, granulated (1 tablespoon)

- Onion, medium, chopped (1 piece)

- Baby lima beans, frozen, thawed, drained (9 ounces)

Directions:

- Preheat air fryer at 325 degrees Fahrenheit.

- Combine all ingredients, save for cheese, in casserole.

- Cover and air-fry for one hour and fifteen minutes. Give dish a stir before topping with cheese.

Nutrition: Calories 440 Fat 6.0 g Protein 20.0 g Carbohydrates 77.0 g

Cheesy Potato Mash Casserole

Preparation time: 25 min

Cooking time: 1 hr 10 min Servings: 24

Ingredients:

- Chives, fresh, chopped (1 teaspoon)

- Cream cheese, reduced fat, softened (3 ounces)

- Yogurt, plain, fat free (1 cup)

- Cheddar cheese, reduced fat, shredded (1 cup)

- Paprika (1/4 teaspoon)

- White potatoes, peeled, cubed (5 pounds)

- Blue cheese, crumbled (1/4 cup)

- Parmesan cheese, shredded (1/4 cup) Garlic salt (1 teaspoon)

Directions:

- Place potatoes in saucepan filled with water. Heat to boiling, then cook on simmer for fifteen to eighteen minutes.

- Beat together parmesan cheese, cheddar cheese, cream cheese, and blue cheese until smooth. Beat in garlic salt and yogurt.

- Preheat air fryer t o 325 degrees Fahrenheit.

- Mash cooked potatoes until smooth. Stir in cheese mixture. Add to a baking dish and air-fry for thirty-five to forty minutes.

Nutrition: Calories 110 Fat 2.5 g Protein 4.0 g Carbohydrates 18.0 g

Simple Squash Casserole

Preparation time: 20 min

Cooking time: 40 min

Servings: 6

Ingredients:

- Yellow summer squash, medium, sliced thinly (1 piece)

- Thyme leaves, fresh, chopped (1 tablespoon)

- Salt (1/2 teaspoon)

- Italian cheese blend, gluten free, shredded (1/2 cup)

- Olive oil, extra virgin (1 tablespoon)

- Zucchini, medium, sliced thinly (1 piece)

- Onion, diced (1/2 cup)

- Brown rice, cooked (1 cup)

- Plum tomato, diced (1 piece) Pepper (1/8 teaspoon)

Directions:

- Preheat air fryer to 375 degrees Fahrenheit.

- Mist cooking spray onto a gratin dish.

- Combine rice, onion, tomato, pepper, salt (1/4 teaspoon), oil, and ½ thyme leaves. Spread evenly into gratin dish and layer on top with squash and zucchini. Sprinkle with remaining salt (1/4 teaspoon) and thyme.

- Cover and air-fry for twenty minutes. Top with cheese and air-fry for another ten to twelve minutes.

Nutrition: Calories 110 Fat 5.0 g Protein 4.0 g Carbohydrates 12.0 g

Delicious Ginger Pork Lasagna

Preparation time: 45 min

Cooking time: 45 min

Servings: 8

Ingredients:

- Thai basil leaves, fresh, sliced thinly (2 tablespoons)

- Butter (1 tablespoon)

- Garlic cloves, minced (2 pieces)

- Ricotta cheese, part skim (15 ounces)

- Wonton wrappers, square (48 pieces)

- Green onion greens & whites, separated, sliced thinly (4 pieces)

- Fish sauce (1 tablespoon)

- Parmesan cheese, shredded (1 tablespoon)

- Sesame oil, toasted (1 tablespoon)

- Ground pork (1 pound)

- Gingerroot, fresh, minced (1 tablespoon)

- Tomato sauce (15 ounces)

- Chili garlic sauce (1 tablespoon) Coconut milk (1/2 cup)

Directions:

- Preheat air fryer at 325 degrees Fahrenheit.

- Mist cooking spray onto a baking dish.

- In skillet heated on medium, cook pork in butter and sesame oil for eight to ten minutes. Stir in garlic, green onion whites, and gingerroot and cook for one to two minutes. Stir in fish sauce, chili garlic sauce, and tomato sauce. Cook on gentle simmer.

- Combine coconut milk, ricotta cheese, and parmesan cheese (1 cup).

- Arrange 8 overlapping wonton wrappers in baking dish to line bottom, then top with a second layer of eight wrappers. Spread on top 1/3 of cheese

- mixture, and layer with 1/3 of pork mixture. Repeat layering twice and finish by topping with parmesan cheese.

- Cover dish with foil and air-fry for thirty minutes. Remove foil and air-fry for another ten to fifteen minutes.

- Serve topped with basil and green onion greens.

Nutrition: Calories 480 Fat 24.0 g Protein 28.0 g Carbohydrates 37.0 g

Baked Sweet Potatoes

Cooking time: 10 minutes

Servings: 2

Ingredients:

- 2 big sweet potatoes, scrubbed

- 1 cup water

- A pinch of salt and black pepper

- ½ teaspoon smoked paprika

- ½ teaspoon cumin, ground

Directions:

- Put the water in your pressure cooker, add the steamer basket, add sweet potatoes inside, cover and cook on High for 10 minutes.

- Split potatoes, add salt, pepper, paprika and cumin, divide them between plates and serve as a side dish.

Nutrition: calories 152, fat 2, fiber 3, carbs 4, protein 4

Broccoli Pasta

Cooking time: 4 minutes

Servings: 2

Ingredients:

- 2 cups water

- ½ pound pasta

- 8 ounces cheddar cheese, grated

- ½ cup broccoli ½ cup half and half

-

Directions:

- Put the water and the pasta in your pressure cooker.

- Add the steamer basket, add the broccoli, cover the cooker and cook on High for 4 minutes.

- Drain pasta, transfer it as well as the broccoli, and clean the pot.

- Set it on sauté mode, add pasta and broccoli, cheese and half and half, stir well, cook for 2 minutes, divide between plates and serve as a side dish for chicken.

Nutrition: calories 211, fat 4, fiber 2, carbs 6, protein 7

Cauliflower Rice

Cooking time: 12 minutes

Servings: 2

Ingredients:

- 1 tablespoon olive oil

- ½ cauliflower head, florets separated

- A pinch of salt and black pepper

- A pinch of parsley flakes

- ¼ teaspoon cumin, ground

- ¼ teaspoon turmeric powder

- ¼ teaspoon paprika

- 1 cup water

- ½ tablespoon cilantro, chopped Juice from 1/3 lime

Directions:

- Put the water in your pressure cooker, add the steamer basket, add cauliflower florets, cover and cook on High for 2 minutes.

- Discard water, transfer cauliflower to a plate and leave aside.

- Clean your pressure cooker, add the oil, set on sauté mode and heat it up. Add cauliflower, mash using a potato masher, add salt, pepper, parsley, cumin, turmeric, paprika, cilantro and lime juice, stir well, cook for 10 minutes more, divide between 2 plates and serve as a side dish.

Nutrition: calories 191, fat 1, fiber 2, carbs 4, protein 5

Refried Beans

Cooking time: 35 minutes

Servings: 2

Ingredients:

- 1 pound pinto beans, soaked for 20 minutes and drained

- 1 cup onion, chopped

- 2 garlic cloves, minced

- 1 teaspoon oregano, dried

- ½ jalapeno, chopped

- 1 teaspoon cumin, ground

- A pinch of salt and black pepper

- 1 and ½ tablespoon olive oil

- 2 cups chicken stock

Directions:

- In your pressure cooker, mix oil with onion, jalapeno, garlic, oregano, cumin, salt, pepper, stock and beans, stir, cover and cook on Manual for 30 minutes.

- Stir beans one more time, divide them between 2 plates and serve as a side dish.

Nutrition: calories 200, fat 1, fiber 3, carbs 7, protein 7

Sweet Brussels Sprouts

Cooking time: 4 minutes

Servings: 2

Ingredients:

- ½ pounds Brussels sprouts

- 2 teaspoon buttery spread

- ½ teaspoon orange zest, grated

- 1 tablespoon orange juice

- ½ tablespoon maple syrup A pinch of salt and black pepper

Directions:

- In your pressure cooker, mix Brussels sprouts with buttery spread, orange zest, orange juice, maple syrup, salt and pepper, stir, cover and cook on High for 4 minutes.

- Divide between 2 plates and serve as a side dish.

Nutrition: calories 65, fat 2, fiber 3, carbs 10, protein 3

Dessert Recipes

Fiesta Pastries

Preparation time: 15 minutes

Cooking time: 20 minutes

Servings: 8

Ingredients:

- ½ of apple, peeled, cored and chopped

- 1 teaspoon fresh orange zest, grated finely

- 7.05-ounce prepared frozen puff pastry, cut into 16 squares

- ½ tablespoon white sugar ½ teaspoon ground cinnamon

Directions:

- Preheat the Air fryer to 390 o F and grease an Air fryer basket.

- Mix all ingredients in a bowl except puff pastry.

- Arrange about 1 teaspoon of this mixture in the center of each square.

- Fold each square into a triangle and slightly press the edges with a fork.

- Arrange the pastries in the Air fryer basket and cook for about 10 minutes. Dish out and serve immediately.

Nutrition:

Calories: 147, Fat: 9.5g, Carbohydrates: 13.8g, Sugar: 2.1g, Protein: 1.9g, Sodium: 62mg

Classic Buttermilk Biscuits

Preparation time: 15 minutes

Cooking time: 8 minutes

Servings: 4

Ingredients:

- ½ cup cake flour

- 1¼ cups all-purpose flour

- ¾ teaspoon baking powder

- ¼ cup + 2 tablespoons butter, cut into cubes

- ¾ cup buttermilk

- 1 teaspoon granulated sugar

- Salt, to taste

Directions:

- Preheat the Air fryer to 400 o F and grease a pie pan lightly.

- Sift together flours, baking soda, baking powder, sugar and salt in a large bowl.

- Add cold butter and mix until a coarse crumb is formed.

- Stir in the buttermilk slowly and mix until a dough is formed.

- Press the dough into ½ inch thickness onto a floured surface and cut out circles with a 1¾-inch round cookie cutter.

- Arrange the biscuits in a pie pan in a single layer and brush butter on them.

- Transfer into the Air fryer and cook for about 8 minutes until golden brown.

Nutrition:

Calories: 374, Fat: 18.2g, Carbohydrates: 45.2g, Sugar: 3.4g, Protein: 7.3g, Sodium: 291mg

Blueberry bowls

Cooking time: 12 minutes

Servings: 4

Ingredients:

- 2 cups blueberries

- cup coconut water

- tablespoons sugar

- 2 teaspoons vanilla extract Juice of ½ lime

Directions:

- In your air fryer's pan, combine the blueberries with the water and the other ingredients, toss and cook at 320 degrees f for 12 minutes.

- Serve cold.

Nutrition: calories 230, fat 2, fiber 2, carbs 14, protein 7

Carrot brownies

Cooking time: 25 minutes

Servings: 8

Ingredients:

- 1 teaspoon almond extract

- 2 eggs, whisked

- ½ cup butter, melted

- 4 tablespoons sugar

- 2 cups almond flour

- ½ cup carrot, peeled and grated

Directions:

- In a bowl, combine the eggs with the butter and the other ingredients, whisk, spread this into a pan that fits your air fryer, introduce in the fryer and cook at 340 degrees f for 25 minutes.

- Cool down, slice and serve.

Nutrition: calories 230, fat 12, fiber 2, carbs 12, protein 5

Yogurt cake

Cooking time: 30 minutes

Servings: 8

Ingredients:

- 6 eggs, whisked

- 1 teaspoon vanilla extract

- 1 teaspoon baking soda

- 9 ounces almond flour

- 4 tablespoons sugar 2 cups yogurt

Directions:

- In a blender, combine the eggs with the vanilla and the other ingredients, pulse, spread into a cake pan lined with parchment paper, put it in the air fryer and cook at 330 degrees f for 30 minutes.

- Cool the cake down, slice and serve.

Nutrition: calories 231, fat 13, fiber 2, carbs 11, protein 5

Chocolate ramekins

Cooking time: 20 minutes

Servings: 4

Ingredients:

- 2 cups cream cheese, soft

- 2 tablespoons sugar

- 3 eggs, whisked

- 1 teaspoon vanilla extract

- ½ cup heavy cream

- 2 cups white chocolate, melted

Directions:

- In a bowl combine the cream cheese with the sugar and the other ingredients, whisk well, divide into 4 ramekins, put them in the air fryer's basket and cook at 370 degrees f for 20 minutes.

- Serve cold.

Nutrition: calories 261, fat 12, fiber 6, carbs 12, protein 6

Grapes cake

Cooking time: 25 minutes

Servings: 8

Ingredients:

- 1 cup coconut flour

- 1 teaspoon baking powder

- ¾ teaspoon almond extract

- ¾ cup sugar

- Cooking spray

- 1 cup heavy cream

- 1 cup grapes, halved1 egg, whisked

Directions:

- In a bowl, combine the flour with the baking powder and the other ingredients except the cooking spray and whisk well.

- Grease a cake pan with cooking spray, pour the cake batter inside, spread, introduce the pan in the air fryer and cook at 330 degrees f for 25 minutes.

- Cool the cake down, slice and serve.

Nutrition: calories 214, fat 9, fiber 3, carbs 14, protein 8

Carrots bread

Cooking time: 40 minutes

Servings: 6

Ingredients:

- 2 cups carrots, peeled and grated

- 1 cup sugar

- 3 eggs, whisked

- 2 cups white flour

- 1 tablespoon baking soda 1 cup almond milk

Directions:

- In a bowl, combine the carrots with the sugar and the other ingredients, whisk well, pour this into a lined loaf pan, introduce the pan in the air fryer and cook at 340 degrees f for 40 minutes.

- Cool the bread down, slice and serve.

Nutrition: calories 200, fat 5, fiber 3, carbs 13, protein 7

Pear pudding

Cooking time: 20 minutes

Servings: 6

Ingredients:

- 3 tablespoons sugar

- ½ cup butter, melted

- 2 eggs, whisked

- 2 pears, peeled and chopped

- 1/3 cup almond milk ½ cup heavy cream

Directions:

- In a bowl, combine the butter with the sugar and the other ingredients, whisk well and pour into a pudding pan.

- Introduce the pan in the air fryer and cook at 340 degrees f for 20 minutes.

- Cool the pudding down, divide into bowls and serve.

Nutrition: calories 211, fat 4, fiber 6, carbs 14, protein 6

Lime cake

Cooking time: 30 minutes

Servings: 4

Ingredients:

- 1 egg, whisked

- 1 tablespoons sugar

- 2 tablespoons butter, melted

- ½ cup almond milk

- 2 tablespoons lime juice

- 1 tablespoon lime zest, grated

- 1 cup heavy cream½ teaspoon baking powder

Directions:

- In a bowl, combine the egg with the sugar, butter and the other ingredients, whisk well and transfer to a cake pan lined with parchment paper.

- Put the pan in your air fryer and cook at 320 degrees f for 30 minutes.

- Serve the cake cold.

Nutrition: calories 213, fat 5, fiber 5, carbs 15, protein 6

Pear stew

Cooking time: 20 minutes

Servings: 4

Ingredients:

- 1 teaspoons cinnamon powder

- 4 pears, cored and cut into wedges

- 1 cup water

- 1 tablespoons sugar

Directions:

- In your air fryer's pan, combine the pears with the water and the other ingredients, cook at 300 degrees f for 20 minutes, divide into cups and serve cold.

Nutrition: calories 200, fat 3, fiber 4, carbs 16, protein 4